Get Ripped Abs!

===============

The Best Way to Get Six-Pack Abs

Ron Kness

ISBN-13: 978-1500909840

ISBN-10: 150090984X

CONTENTS

INTRODUCTION

We are enthralled with six-pack abs. In the fitness world, having a set seems to be the ultimate visual evidence of a fit body. People go to great lengths to try and get "washboard" abs, but few succeed. Why is that?

The truth is we all have the same abdominal muscles, so if fact we all have six-pack abs. But having them and being able to see them can be two very different things.

The focus of this book is to show you what you can do with your abs to work them, define them and make them come through visually, so that when you rip off your shirt, people take notice.

Every single person has a six-pack, just the same as every single person has a pair of biceps. What you might not know is that many factors go into the shaping and defining them, just like biceps.

One of the factors is genetics – not something you can change. You are stuck with your basic body shape. You can't appreciably change that any more than you can change your height. For people that tend to carry less fat around their mid-section, it is quicker for them to get to a point where their abs are visible; if you carry more body fat in the midsection, you'll have to work harder to make your abs come through.

Make no mistake about it, belly fat is tough to get rid of. That's why to many people having a six-pack is the ultimate goal when it comes to fitness because whenever you are losing weight, belly fat is the last thing to disappear before your abs can appear.

Despite what you may have read or heard, spot reducing is not possible. The body just doesn't work that way. When you lose body fat, it comes off from all parts of the body, although not equally. Belly fat is one of the last places to lose as it is the deepest fat. Fat loss starts at the surface and works its way deeper into the body.

While you care how you look (or you wouldn't be reading this book), your body doesn't. Through evolution, your body developed a sense of survival. In lean times when not much food is available, it goes into starvation mode burning as few calories as possible to "weather the storm" until food is again plentiful.

Your body wants that layer of fat to use as an energy source should the need arise. That is also one of the factors that make losing body fat so difficult – you are working against what your body has been evolutionized to do – conserve fat.

As we said earlier, the reason that everyone doesn't have visible abs depends on a variety of factors. We talked about one factor being genetics. Other factors include:

- not exercising regularly

- eating the wrong foods and too much of it

- and in some people, not having the desire to change.

However, regardless what anyone says or tries to tell you, you do have abs, now it's up to you and the help of this guide to transform them into a six-pack. Whether or not you decide put in the work, and take the time to reveal them is up to you.

As the old saying goes "You can lead a horse to water, but you can't make 'em drink." In this book I lead you to the water. It's up to you to decide if you want to drink or not.

Chapter 1 – Can I Get Six-Pack Abs?

The short answer is yes! But it isn't easy. One thing you have to realize is for you to have a visible six-pack you have to reach a certain body fat percentage – around 10% for men and 17% for women.

You can increase the definition of your abs by doing exercises designed to tone and increase the size of your abs, but if you are still carrying too much body fat, nobody will see them.

So to have visible abs you first have to reduce your body fat. For right now, this is key. Once the body fat is down, then we'll switch gears and focus on building out the abs.

From here we will go into the changes in diet and exercising that you'll have to make to get your body fat down. For those carrying more body fat, this will be harder and take longer, but know that it is within reach of everyone. The secrets are consistency and determination; starting the program and committing to staying on it and the drive to get right back on that horse again when you fall off your diet and/or exercise program (and fall off you will – most likely multiple times).

There are many factors that go into weight loss, but a good place to start are calories consumed verses calories burned. You are eating a certain number of calories each day and I assume you are maintaining your weight right now – not gaining or losing an appreciable amount.

So to lose weight, you have to burn more calories than you consume or consume fewer calories than you burn – depending on how you look at it.

Either way, to lose one pound of weight per week, you have to have a 3,500 calorie deficit during that week. While that may seem insurmountable, when you break it down into a 500-calorie-per-day deficit, it is more manageable.

For example, if you switch from drinking a couple of full strength sodas – one having real sugars – to a couple of diet sodas, you've cut out 280 calories or more. Add in one cardio exercise for 30 minutes, such as brisk walking, and a 180-pound person burns around 198 calories. Just these two small changes and you are almost at your 500-calorie-per-day deficit.

The truth is that everyone can develop their abs. The variable is how long it will take. Some people always seem to have abs regardless of what they do or eat. For other people, it is going to take a lot of work, and it is going to be frustrating. Like with most anything else training related, consistency is the key to success – both in diet and exercise. If you stay consistent and monitor all the aspects of your training and diet, you can build an awesome set of abs that ripple down your front.

Chapter 2 – Considerations When Starting an Ab Training Program

Training your abs is no different than training any other muscle. If you want results you have to create a plan and you have to put forth consistent effort.

Another thing to consider with ab training is that you have to be patient. The abs are always the last thing to reveal themselves, so it makes sense that they will take the most time to develop.

3 Things to Consider When Beginning Ab Training

- It's going to take longer than you expect

- It's going to be harder than you thought

- You are going to have to eat healthy and in the proper quantities

It cannot be overemphasized that getting a six-pack is really hard work. Part of the problem is there are so many infomercials out there that tell you that you can have a six-pack in 8 weeks. And for those that don't have much body fat to lose, it is possible. However for the rest of us, it is going to take longer.

The biggest challenge to start with is setting a goal. Be careful with this and remember a goal has to be realistic and attainable. Getting a six-pack in 8 weeks is most likely neither.

The problem is that when you set unrealistic and unattainable expectations, chances are you will fail. And when you fail to reach your goal, you are likely to get frustrated and give up. Once you give up the first time it gets harder and harder to start again because you expect to fail again.

A more realistic and attainable goal to get a six-pack would be "to control my calorie intake to 1,800 calories per day, cardio train 4 days per week and do strength training 2 days per week for 30 minutes each time." This entirely doable and if you stick to your regimen, you should lose 1 to 1.5 pounds of weight per week. Just be sure your calorie goal is appropriate for you and don't accept the 1,800 calories I used as gospel. Your calorie needs may be different. To find out what your requirements are use this calorie calculator from the Mayo Clinic.

Besides the time factor another thing to consider is lower back training. As with all your training you want to make sure your physique is balanced. If you significantly increase your ab training without increasing your lower back training, you will develop muscular imbalances. This is a recipe for disaster and can lead to lower back issues or injury. Take this into consideration when you plan your training.

The bottom line is before you have any visions of washboard abs and start to train abs, be realistic about how long it is going to take and balance out your training. Just realize it is going to take longer than you think and it is going to be more work anticipate, but in the end the pay-off will be worth it!

Once you reach your goal you will have a sense of accomplishment, and an awesome six-pack too.

Chapter 3 – Eating Right to Get Six-Pack Abs

As important as training is, when it comes to abs, diet is more important. By some estimates, diet is 70% of the equation, exercising 30%.

No other muscle group is as dependent on diet as the abs, because abs only appear once your body fat percentage is down. While it is true that you can build the abs to be more visible, you still are going to have to drop body fat to have them show through the way you want them to.

In this chapter, we are going to look at 5 nutrition tips for six-pack abs:

- Eliminate sugar

- Increase protein consumption

- Eat healthy fats

- Eat whole unprocessed foods

- Drinks lots of water

Eliminate sugar – Pretty much every piece of diet advice will tell you to reduce or eliminate sugar intake. This list is obviously no exception. The main problem with sugar is that it is a simple carbohydrate that digests quickly causing an insulin spike.

Once insulin levels spike, fat burning comes to a halt because your body wants to eat through that sugar as fast as possible, so it uses it as the primary source of energy until it is gone. If you want your body to be a fat burning machine then you have to keep blood sugar levels steady and reduce the effects of insulin. That is not to say that you have to avoid carbs altogether. As a matter-of-fact you have to have carbohydrates present in order to burn fat; just make sure they are complex carbs which take longer to breakdown. A quality post-workout shake with carbs in it is a good way to replenish glycogen in the muscle and help you recover.

Increase protein consumption – While you do need a caloric deficit to lose weight, you don't want to lose the muscle in the process.

If you are lowering carb intake, then you have to get those calories from somewhere else. Consuming protein in the form of lean cuts of meat is optimal. Protein shakes are convenient, but it is better to get most of your calories from whole foods.

Drinking your calories does not give you the same level of satisfaction, and being in a caloric deficit is hard enough. Also there is a thermogenic effect - heat generated by the digestion process - that you do not get when you drink your calories.

Eat healthy fats – No matter what you may hear, low fat diets are ineffective. Your body needs good healthy fats – the Omegas and unsaturated.

You also have to consider that the more fat you consume (up to a point), the more efficient you become at processing it. If you reduce your fat intake then your body does not produce as many fat burning enzymes. So you should include healthy fats in your meal plans. Just pay attention to your calories as fats are very calorie dense – 9 calories per gram compared with 4 each for carbs and protein.

Eat whole unprocessed foods – This is good advice whether you want abs or not. Both from a health and dieting standpoint, it is best to consume unprocessed foods. These foods have more nutritional value, and when you are reducing calories you need the most nutrient dense foods you can find.

Drinks lots of water – Hydration is important whether you are dieting or not. However, when you are dieting it can help for numerous reasons. Drinking lots of water helps you feel full and reduces hunger cravings. In fact the more water that you drink, the more water you excrete. You can reduce your water retention by drinking more water, and the less water sloshing around inside of you, the more visible your abs will be.

None of these suggestions are particularly exciting. In fact you will probably find these on every diet tips list you ever read. There is a reason for that; they work. People are always looking for short cuts to dieting and getting abs, but there aren't any. It still comes down to eating fewer calories and burning more through exercising.

If you concentrate on these two basics, you'll see your abs sooner and have more money in your pocket because you didn't buy all the things you see in infomercials that make losing weight easy; they don't exist.

Chapter 4 – Taking Your Eating to the Next Level to Get Six-Pack Abs

There are a lot of factors when it comes to building six-pack abs. Some of them, like genetics, are beyond your control. However, training and diet are two things you can control.

Make no mistake about it ab training is very important. However, your dream of abs lives and dies with your diet. Remember in the last chapter we said 70% of the weight loss equation was diet?

You can do all the work you want in the gym, and completely sabotage your results in the kitchen. Or as experts say "You can't exercise your way out of a bad diet." Since abs are the last to appear and the first to disappear, diet will always play a huge part in how your six-pack looks. The message here is once you get a six-pack, you'll have to go on an eating and exercise maintenance program to keep them visible.

How restrictive you have to be in regards to diet depends on many things. However, just when you might start to think it is impossible to get your six-pack, there is good news. There are actually super foods that can help speed up the fat loss process and bring your abs out for the entire world to see sooner.

5 Super Foods for Six-Pack Abs

- Whole Eggs

- Grass Fed Butter

- Grass Fed Beef

- Wild Fish

- Dark Leafy Greens

Whole Eggs – You might not expect eggs to be on this list, they are an excellent source of protein. They have a very impressive amino acid profile, and they offer good fats. Eggs will not only help with fat loss, but they will help you build muscle. This is a one-two punch when it comes to building a six-pack. It is important to note that when it comes to eggs you should be eating free range organic. And don't worry about the yolk; it is good for you too.

Grass Fed Butter – I am sure you think that butter will make you fat. The truth it is depends on the type of butter. Grass fed butter is one of the best sources of conjugated linoleic acid (CLA). CLA has been shown to not only help with weight loss, but increase your resistance to carcinogens. Not only that, but it has a great ratio of Omega 3 to Omega 6 fatty acids.

Grass Fed Beef – Much like butter, grass fed beef has many more health benefits than your average feed lot raised beef. It has been shown to have 10 times the beta-carotene, three times the Vitamin E and 3 times the Omega 3 fatty acids.

Wild Fish – We all know that fish oil is a powerful supplement, and that we eat far too much Omega 6 and not enough Omega 3. Wild caught fish are full of healthy Omega 3's as well as being high in protein. Salmon, halibut, mackerel and tuna are the ones highest in Omega 3.

Dark Leafy Greens – When it comes to six-pack abs, Popeye was right. The dark leafy greens, such as spinach, kale, and bok choy, are perfect super foods for your six-pack plans. They help you reach your nutritional requirements, and are great sources of vitamins and minerals, and have very few calories. They are nutrient dense foods and when you are dieting that is a necessity.

I hope this list of superfoods helps in your awareness of super foods that can have a big impact on your diet and play a big part in revealing those six-pack abs.

Chapter 5 – Top Supplements to Get Six-Pack Abs

We cannot get away from the fact that diet has a huge impact on our quest for six-pack abs. What you eat (or not eat) has a huge impact on your results.

The supplement industry knows this, and makes billions of dollars each year selling you quick fix solutions to your body fat problems. Unfortunately most of the supplements out there do nothing to help you attain your goal.

But with that said, there are some supplements that have stood the test of time. People spend too much time looking for the latest and greatest shortcut to help them lose weight overnight - stop looking because it doesn't exist. However, to help speed up the weight loss/ muscle building process here are some solid supplement choices.

5 Best Supplements for Six-pack Abs:

- Caffeine
- CLA

- Yohimbe

- Synephrine

- Green Tea

Caffeine – Not only does your morning coffee help you wake up in the morning; it aids in fat loss. Caffeine is a CNS stimulant that binds to fat and enhances fat burning. Unfortunately your body can become immune to your normal caffeine dose so it may be necessary to cycle on and off from time to time to get the same effect. And in reality, your morning cup of joe is not the best way to get caffeine. Go with capsules in 100mg size. Usually two capsule an hour before exercising produces the best results.

CLA – Conjugated linoleic acid is a healthy fat that is a true powerhouse when it comes to six-pack abs. It has been shown to boost strength, shred body fat and build muscle. CLA actually blocks certain fat storing enzymes, thus preventing the storage of fat.

Yohimbe – You will find Yohimbe in most fat burning stacks. Its effects are well documented. It works in a different method from other fat burners in that it blocks the alpha receptors on fat cells. Yohimbe can be taken orally, or if you find it in a cream form you can apply it directly to the ab area.

Synephrine – We all know the caffeine, ephedrine and aspirin stack worked well for fat loss. Unfortunately ephedrine is no longer available. Synephrine has a similar chemical structure to ephedrine, but it increases fat burning without increasing your heart rate or raising your blood pressure.

Green Tea – Green tea contains catechins. EGCG is the main catechin, in green tea and it is responsible for the thermogenic effects produced from drinking green tea. EGCG works to inhibit norepinephrine break down, which allows you to maintain a high level of calorie burning.

This might not be an exciting list, but the truth is these supplements work.

You can waste your time with the latest and greatest, or you can stick to the basics. There is a reason these supplements have been around forever. Add them to your mix and you will see an increase in your results.

Chapter 6 – An Exercise Routine for Fast Results

So you have your diet under control and are ready to start your journey towards six-pack abs. The problem is you have no idea what you should do. Here is a sample routine that is a good place to start. Remember it is important when you are just starting out to learn proper exercise technique. Any bad habits you learn in the beginning will tend to stick with you, so if you need help, just Google the exercise and lots of options will come up that you can use.

Beginner's Ab Workout

- Cable Ab Pull downs - 3 sets of 15 repetitions in each set

- Straight Leg Raises - 3 sets of 15 repetitions in each set

- Hyperextension Side Bends - 3 sets of 15 repetitions in each set

- Ab Wheel - 2 sets of 20 repetitions in each set

Once you can easily complete the all repetitions in the exercise, add weight and that will drop you back as far as the number of repetitions you can do before muscle failure. Keep using this add-weight strategy to keep your body burning calories and adding muscle mass.

<u>Cable Ab Pulldown</u> – This is one of the best ab exercises because it allows you to use train the abs while standing.

Lying on the ground and training your abs is very unnatural, you need to learn to contract your abs while standing. For this exercise you need a cable machine with a high pulley and a triceps rope.

Starting position for this exercise is standing facing away from the machine. Take the handles and pull them down around the sides of your neck so you can hold them against your chest. From there you perform a standing crunch until your upper body is perpendicular to the floor; then return to an upright position. To get the full benefit from the exercise, also resist and come back up slowly.

Lying Straight Leg Raises – Lay on a weight bench or exercise mat. Place hands under you lower buttocks on each side to support the pelvis. Keeping your knees straight, raise your legs by flexing at the hips until your feet are point toward the ceiling. Lower your legs until your legs are extended and parallel with the floor. Repeat.

Hyperextension Side Bends – On a 45-degree hyperextension bench, begin by standing sideways. Make sure the pad is properly placed against your hip, and lower that side of yourself down towards the floor.

When your upper body is parallel to the floor, contract your obliques hard as you return to your starting position. This is an exercise that you can progressively add weight to by using a dumbbell in the hand closest to the floor, a weight plate against your chest, or a weight plate behind your head.

Ab Wheel – This basic exercise is often overlooked, but it is very effective. It is basically an ab plank with movement added.

Simply kneel on the floor, and grip the handles of the wheel in front of you. Slowly roll out as far as you can, and then contract your abs as you pull yourself back to the starting position. Once you have gotten the hang of it you can roll out to either side too instead of just a straight line for added variety and to work your abs a little differently.

Chances are if you are consistent you will quickly outgrow this workout. However when you are just starting out, it is always a good idea to keep it simple. Obviously there are many more advanced techniques that you will learn as your progress, but this routine is a good place for you to start.

For many people ab training just means lying on the floor and doing crunches. They think that if they just do 1,000 crunches a day, they will have six-pack abs in no time flat.

Who can blame them since they are constantly shown commercials for workouts promising just that?

Unfortunately we all know that is not true. To really build a six-pack you have to mix up your exercises and hit the abs from different angles. That is not to say that crunches should not be in your exercise routine, because they should; we're saying they shouldn't be your only exercise.

Once you are ready for more advanced crunches, try adding in these ab exercises to your routine:

- Bicycle Crunches

- Reverse Crunches

Bicycle Crunches – Often times when it comes to ab training, we only work in one plane. However the abs are built to perform in numerous planes.

Adding some twisting to your ab exercises is a great way to stimulate new muscles like the oblique and serratus. For a demonstration, click on the Bicycle Crunches link.

Reverse Crunches – We spend so much time focusing on the upper abs that we often forget about the lower abs. This imbalance can cause a number of problems. Besides building a midsection that is not symmetrical, you are setting yourself up for an injury. While ab muscles are very resistant to injury, if you happen to pull one you will remember it forever. Here again, click the link for a demonstration video of how to do reverse crunches.

This is just a short list of ab exercises to help add some variety to your training. If you need any help with how to perform the exercise or technique, just click on the links provided.

Don't get stuck in the rut of thinking that crunches are the only thing you can do. You have to mix it up in order to keep your body growing. Not incorporation variety in your workout will eventually stagnate your progress or allow yourself to get bored. If you stick with your plan, you will eventually reach your six-pack goal.

Chapter 7 – Cardio Train for Six-Pack Abs

For some reason when people want six-pack abs the first thing they think is that they just need to do a little more cardio and they will get there. Obviously diet and other training aspects factor into the equation and cardio does have its place in your six-pack ab training; you just have to be careful not to overdo it.

Some people can become obsessed with getting their six-pack, which isn't necessarily bad. However, when that obsession leads to them doing hours and hours of cardio a week it can be a problem.

When you put yourself in too great of a caloric deficit your body will have no choice but to burn muscle. While you will be losing weight, that weight will be muscle and you continue to get softer and softer.

When it comes to cardio for your six-pack, less is often better. If your diet and training are on point then you don't need to go crazy with your cardio. In fact if your cardio is intense enough you could get away with doing only an hour a week or so.

HIIT Cardio for Six-pack Abs

If you have never heard of HIIT it stands for High Intensity Interval Training. It consists of doing a short duration of really intense exercise followed by a longer duration of lower intensity exercise. For the sake of cardio, it might involve sprinting for 20-30 seconds and then walking for 90 seconds to 2 minutes and then sprinting again. Or sprinting on a bike or rowing machine or whatever form of cardio that you can give an all-out effort for a short period of time and then drop down to a lesser intensity.

HIIT cardio is the best bet cardio for fat loss. With HIIT you hit your muscles hard with short, intense workouts that burn the maximal amount of fat. Not only that, but you continue to burn fat after your workout - at a much higher rate than traditional slow steady cardio. A couple of HIIT sessions a week is all you need. It is much more effective and efficient than spending 45 minutes a day on a treadmill.

Keep in mind that cardio is mainly for burning fat, while weight or strength training is for building muscle.

Chapter 8 – Pitfalls to Avoid Along the Way

So many people want six-pack abs, but very few people have them. Have you ever wondered why that is? The truth is that many people train their abs incorrectly and consequently, get poor results. Those poor results lead to them giving up. So how can you avoid making the same mistakes that they are making? Learn from them by not making these same five training mistakes:

- Doing too many crunches

- Not enough intensity

- Not actually training abs

- Only training upper abs

- Trying to crunch out of a poor diet

Doing too many crunches – Crunches are a great exercise for six-pack abs, but they aren't the only exercise. Too often people fall into the trap of just doing crunches, and obviously this is far from optimal. Your abs are made up of numerous different muscles, they move in different direction, and in different planes. You have to constantly hit them from different angles to get results.

Not enough intensity – For some reason people think that high reps are the only way to train abs. This simply is not true. As noted earlier we showed that HIIT is a short duration but high intensity way to train.

Your abs respond to training just like any other training, and constantly doing sets of 50 is not always the best way to go. You need to vary your intensity of your ab work just like you would any other muscle group. In fact you should focus on training to grow your abs instead of just toning them. It is almost impossible for your abs to get too big, so mix in some high intensity techniques and get them growing.

Not actually training abs – This actually happens more than you might think. Some people think that they can just diet and cardio their way to a six-pack.

Other people try to work their abs, but miss the mark. They end up spending the majority of their ab workout hitting their hip flexors and aggravating their spinal erectors. If you want six-pack abs you have to actually train your abs, and you have to train them correctly. Make sure the exercises you are doing are actually one that are meant to work your abs.

Only training upper abs – This is similar to the above mentioned mistake. You have to understand that the abs consist of much more than just the upper rectus abdominis. The truth is there are 4 ab areas to train.

The other 3 include the lower rectus abdominis, the obliques, and the transverse abdominis. When you train your abs and only hit the upper abs it is similar to training your arms and only doing biceps. For complete development you have to hit all the ab muscles.

Trying to crunch out of a poor diet – This is one that many people fall prey to. They think that they can have a bad diet, and if they just work hard enough they will still have a six-pack. Unfortunately this just isn't true. There is a saying that you can't out train a bad diet, and it is very true.

Yes you build your abs in the gym, but you help remove the fat that is covering them in the kitchen.

While there are more mistakes that can be made when it comes to ab training, these seem to be the most common. If you concentrate on avoiding them, your ab training will be well ahead of the game. With consistent, intelligent ab training, you can get the six-pack you want.

Chapter 9 – Maintaining Your Abs

If you are one of the few people that have built an impressive set of abs you now face an even bigger challenge. How do I maintain my six-pack year round? Thankfully ab maintenance is slightly easier than digging them out from underneath the fat to begin with....but not by much.

Society is always trying to sabotage your results with poor food choices or excuses to skip the gym altogether. Here are some tips to help you keep your abs all year:

- Make smart decisions

- Be prepared

- Avoid stress

- Schedule cheat days

- Work for your carbs

Make smart decisions – This can apply to any goal that you have, but when it comes to abs you have to understand that every choice has a consequence. Usually it comes down to food choices, but this can also apply to skipping a training day. You have to ask yourself if the decision you are about to make gets you closer to your goal or not. If not, you either have to rethink your decision or accept the consequence.

Be prepared – Whenever you are away from your own kitchen, poor food choices are waiting to surprise you around every corner. Social gatherings and peer pressure are a great way for you to lose your abs. So always have healthy alternatives available. And depending on the situation sometimes that is not possible. In those cases, decide to make the best decision of what will hurt you the least and drive on.

Avoid stress – We all know that excessive stress causes cortisol to be released into the bloodstream. If your cortisol levels are constantly elevated it will stimulate fat storage. This obviously is a death sentence for your abs, so try to avoid excessive stress at all costs.

Schedule cheat days – When trying to maintain your abs, you are going to always have to watch what you eat. Over the course of a year that can lead up to a lot of frustration. So rather than risk getting fed up and give into your craving by binging (and then feeling guilty about it later), it is best to schedule cheat days where you can eat what you want in moderation. Not only does this means you always have something to look forward to, but it keeps your craving in check by intelligently giving into them once a week.

Work for your carbs – We all love carbs, but the insulin response they cause can wreak havoc on our abs. You don't have to deprive yourself of them, but you should always make sure you earn them. Make sure you are consistently burning enough calories to warrant eating them.

One thing you must realize is that your body doesn't care if your abs are visible or not. In fact it would prefer if you carried an extra layer of fat to help ensure survival.

To maintain abs year round you are going to have to have a plan, and stick to it. You can allow yourself an occasional liberty, but if you ease up too much your abs will go back into hiding.

Conclusion– Action Plan for Six-Pack Abs

So you are ready to uncover your abs and you want to get started right away. The truth is there are a lot of variables when it comes to six-pack ab training. It is best not to get in too much of a hurry, and to make sure all your bases are covered.

At the same time there is no time like the present to start working towards your fitness goals. Here is a five-tip ab action plan to get your started today towards the six-pack you've always dreamed of:

- Set your goal

- Set your timeline

- Structure your diet

- Decide on checkpoints along the way

- Get started

Set Your Goal – Ok we know your goal is a six-pack, but you have to visualize exactly what that is. At what level will you be satisfied? You have to know how far you want to go before you decide on how you will get there. A good idea would be to find someone whose physique you admire and want to aspire to. Then cut it out or save it to your desktop and everyday spend a moment to look at it and visualize your body looking like that.

Set Your Timeline – You have to be realistic when it comes to how long it will take. Think about how long it took to gain all that extra weight in the first place. Get all those "8-weeks-to-abs" infomercials out of your head. You have to understand that getting a six-pack, and then maintaining it, is going to be a long term thing. If you set an unrealistic timeline you are likely to get frustrated and quit.

Structure Your Diet – We all know that most of the work for a six-pack is done in the kitchen. You have to make sure that your diet is on point. More importantly you have to make sure it is right for you specifically. Just taking a diet off of a website won't guarantee success. You have to learn what foods, in what quantities work for you specifically.

Decide on Checkpoints Along the Way – Your long term goal is a six-pack, but it is important to have planned checkpoints along the way. Whether it is weight loss or waist circumference you need to constantly monitor your progress to make sure you are on track. If you are not, then you need to change something.

Get Started – Don't wait around until everything is perfect. There never will be a perfect time to start. Just decide to start today. The more time you spend working towards your goal of a six-pack, the more you will learn about yourself. The best way to figure this all out is by doing it. So don't put this off, and don't wait any longer.

Clearly there is much more to ab training than this, but this is a good place to start. Everyone reacts differently to things and you will constantly have to monitor your progress to see what you need to change. One important thing, if what you are doing isn't working, change it. Don't keep doing the same thing over and over and expect different results.

There is an old saying that goes something like this "If you keep doing the same thing, you'll keep getting the same results."At the same time don't change everything at once, or you won't know which change made the difference.

Well that brings us to an end of our beginners guide to revealing your six-pack abs. I'm glad we've been able to take this journey towards six-pack abs together, all the best with it and start today!

About the Author

I grew up in Central Minnesota, where my parents own and operated a fishing resort. Once out of high school I tried a couple of semesters of college, only to quit halfway through the Spring term; I decided at that time that college wasn't for me.

Then I decided to follow my father's previous occupation as an auto mechanic. I graduated from a two-year of vocational training course and worked as a mechanic. While in vocational training, I decided to join the National Guard where I eventually ended up working full-time for 32 years.

So how does all of this relate to writing? In one of my leadership schools, the instructor, who was an English teacher at a juvenile detention center, presented writing to me in a whole new way - a way that started to develop my interest in working with words.

Fast forward about 40 years and I now have over 20 books listed on Amazon.